I0425110

DIARY OF A PHAT CHICK

J. CAMILLE KELLY

Diary of a Phat Chick

DEDICATION

Everyone says you're supposed to love yourself no matter what size and I do but, when I was headed towards 300lbs I couldn't lose the weight and decided to chronicle my year after surgery to help others get a gastric bypass, an operation I knew would change my life. I have going thru the journey. I relied on my family to see me thru the journey and to be my support group.

To my big sister Sara whose support made my journey easier? She took me into her home and encouraged me more than she realizes .A special thanks for my nephew Quency who made my protein shakes and reminded me to take my vitamins daily. For my niece Zyleah whose help and support during my recovery was appreciated. Special For my niece Ziane, my shopping companion who shopped with me without complaining. To Vanessa my telephone therapist, who had the procedure herself and was always available to lend an ear and share her own journey. To all my friends who watched me take the journey and prayed for my recovery. I love you all. To the little ones, Josslyn, Ricky, Taylor, J'Nei, and Amani thanks for the laughter.

PROLOGUE

My weight loss journey began in January when I decided to have surgery. I don't know what made me decide to have surgery. I guess that I was sick and tired of being fat. I felt depressed and a long term relationship I had had ended the previous year after over 10 years of off and on back and forth and infidelity. I was at a loss as to what to do with myself. I was getting older and I knew that I had a family history of high blood pressure and diabetes. (My mother died of a heart attack) I consumed sweets more than fruits and vegetables. I was a binge eater. I could eat whole cheesecakes in a day. Of course you feel guilty the next day but I had to satisfy the craving and the need to eat to fill the emptiness I was feeling. I already had high blood pressure and took two medications. While having a stressful job it was a matter of time when I would have a stroke so I knew that I had to change my life. I consulted my medical doctor who referred me to a bariatric surgeon. My medical doctor had to write a letter for the health insurance company to prove that I needed the surgery for health reasons and I was 100 pounds overweight. Next I had to make an appointment with the bariatric surgeon for a consultation. When I met with Dr. Silva he was an older doctor and he but me at ease and informed me that I would lose about 80 pounds but that the risk with any surgery is death. I was willing to go the distance and there was no turning back now. When I make up my mind to do something that's it I am focused on the outcome and I get tunnel vision. Dr. Silva explained that it would take about 6 months to complete the testing I needed before surgery. I had to have a stress test, which consisted of me running on a treadmill, and then they measure your heart rate, I had a gastrointestinal test, which they put you to sleep and then put a tub down your throat to see what I do not know. I also saw a psychiatrist, which asked me only if I understood what the operation was about and to see if I had any exaggerated expectations about the results. He talked to me for about 10 minutes to determine my mental stability for the surgery. Who was he kidding, how could I be mentally stabile and be willing to do this to my body not knowing what the results would be or knowing that I might not even survive the surgery.

<u>DECEMBER 12, 2006</u>

I was really going to do this! It was the day before my surgery. I felt a little nervous but there was no turning back now. I was fat and it was time to face the music. I was not fabulous. I was not healthy. I was no longer comfortable in my skin. I loved me but not the fat me. I was tired of shopping at the only two clothing stores for large women. I needed change in my life. I wanted a new life. My mother had passed away two years ago and I still felt like I was walking in a daze some days. I need to snap back and get back into the world. It's been about three years since I have had a real date. I had forgotten what sex was and I had no special person in my life.

I decided to spend my last fat day with my oldest sister and her kids ages 2 and 5 so that she could go out because it was her birthday. I tried to decide what would be my last meal and what I would miss most. My favorite food is pizza and cheesecake from the

Cheesecake Factory, especially vanilla bean. Oh, how I would miss this but it would be worth it. I would now be forced to eat in moderation.

For breakfast I ate three brown and serve sausages and two eggs. Lunch was tuna and white rice. I love the way my sister cooks white rice it doesn't need any seasonings or gravy. I had the same for dinner. I love tuna fish. Since I decided to have my surgery before Christmas, friends asked me about missing the holiday foods. My reply was no because to me Thanksgiving is my big holiday to eat. For me Christmas was just another day. I have no children and the celebration has lost something for me since my grandmother died sixteen years ago two weeks before Christmas. (You never get over the death of a loved one.) I will miss eggnog and sugar cookies on Christmas Eve but how many years have I done this, a change is needed. My sister brought me some chocolates with liquor inside but I only had a couple because I'm not a big drinker, I won't miss liquor.

DECEMBER 13, 2006

The big day was here!!!! I had not eaten or drank anything for 12 hours. When I arrived about 10 am, I was taken care of immediately because someone had cancelled his or her surgery. The anesthesiologist came to talk to me and then gave me a needle to deaden my hand before they inserted a six-inch big thick needle into my hand.

I couldn't believe that they were going to put that needle into my hand. I wanted to run but there was no turning back now. After all the room was reserved. A nurse came and had me walk into the operating room and I was asleep before the doctor came into the room. I don't know if my doctor did the surgery or not. I was having the old fashion Bariatric surgery, where they cut your stomach about 4-6 inches and open you up and make you a smaller stomach about the size of an egg. Next they sewed me up on the inside and put stables on the outside of my stomach. Subsequently, the next thing I heard was a nurse calling my name to wake up and I just wanted to sleep. I know from prior surgery that you have to be awakened in recovery before they take you to a room to go to sleep. I love the euphoria of an induced sleep. I was not feeling any pain. I was wheeled to my room on a stretcher. When I got to my room I recall that there were about four persons trying to put me in bed. I felt groggy and just wanted them to lift me up.

Hello, you're almost 300 pounds!!! I had to move from the stretcher to the bed myself. They do this much easier on T.V. When I woke up, I noticed that it was dark outside but I only wanted to sleep more. However, during the night, someone came to take my blood at an ungodly hour and interrupted my sleep again. I drifted in and out sleep for hours not fully feeling as though I had had enough sleep.

DECEMBER 14, 2006

The first day after surgery I awoke and felt some pain but I had a morphine drip, which I could, self-administer as needed for pain but for me that was as often as I could. I liked the euphoria of a drug-induced sleep.

My morning began with the attending doctor coming around with a group of about six interns to check on me. I felt like the sideshow freak as I lifted my gown so they could see the fat girl's wounds. The interns looked embarrassed just like me but it was part of their training and they were gracious.

After they left I began my regiment of liquids. The breakfast tray came and included apple juice, cranberry juice, and hot water for tea. I had to drink two ounces of juice every thirty minutes. I mixed half the cranberry juice and diluted it with water because my nutritionist had warned that too much sugar would result in stomach pain and diarrhea. Every half hour I drank it was filling and tiring at the same time. I just lay there and watched the clock every thirty minutes to stay on my routine. It was the same menu for breakfast, lunch and dinner.

When one of the nurses came to me and said that I would have to get out of the bed and sit in the chair tomorrow. I was tired and thought that she was crazy. I had a catheter in my vagina and just wanted to sleep and be left alone. You don't get a lot of rest in the hospital.

My girlfriend came to see me in the hospital. She wanted to know that I was all right and being taken care of. I looked horrible but the operation had gone well and I was alive. My face was so dry that it was white. My hair wasn't combed and I had no strength to care about either right now. My nails were done. I routinely get my nails done every two weeks.

<u>DECEMBER 15, 2006</u>

I woke dreading the day that I would have to get out of bed. I felt sluggish and I had never felt so drowsy and listless. I had no energy and the doctor wanted me to get out of bed. I just wanted to lie in bed and heal. However, that's not the way it goes. A male nurse helped me out of bed into the chair alone and without a problem.

Where was he when I first came in to get me from the stretcher to the bed? He was strong and very manly. I sat in the chair and watched television. It felt strange to sit up but I knew that I had to get myself together if I wanted to go home.

A nurse's assistant provided me with some water and soap to wash up because I could not get into the shower. I guess I must have smelled. But, have you ever been so tired and weak that you just didn't care. I felt tired and listless and did not want to wash. I fell asleep in the chair after an hour but continued to sit there for about five or six hours until a nurse helped me back to bed.

A voice in my head said you have to get it together so you can go home. I needed to care about how I looked so I called my niece Zyleah to bring me some lotion for my dry skin and she did. Now I don't have to have a dried up face anymore.

DECEMBER 16, 2006

I started to feel better today but my blood pressure was elevated. I found out when they came around to do vitals, which they do every time a shift changes. They wake you up for this too. When the doctor came around today with his interns he examined my stomach and exposed me to the group of doctors again. This was not a pleasant feeling having about six or more people stare at you, but I smiled and allowed it. The doctor informed me that I would have to consume four ounces every hour and move my bowels before I could go home. Two ounces every half hour was filling. How could I do four ounces? The voice within said you can do it and you have to if you want to go home. Later the nurse came to remove the catheter so I would have to walk to the bathroom. Where they crazy? I couldn't make it to the bathroom with all the liquids I was consuming. Making it across the room to the bathroom was harder than you could imagine. It was like walking down a long hallway and the more you walk the farther away it gets.

When the catheter came out I realized that my period had come when I wet the bed and saw the blood. I called the nurse to come and change the bed then I called my niece and asked her to bring me some Depends because I couldn't make it to the bathroom without pissing on myself half the time. The doctor wanted me to walk and get out of bed and didn't want me in depends but I couldn't make it without them. Between my period and my not being able to make it to the bathroom I was getting frustrated and had second thoughts about what I had done to my body.

I was able to take a shower today after I had a bowel movement. Of course I didn't make it to the bathroom and there were some droppings on the floor from my bed to the bathroom. I called the nurse who called maintenance to clean up the mess.

I was tired of being in the hospital and after four days I wanted out of the hospital. I was drinking my four ounces, had a bowel movement and was up and walking. LET ME OUT! Was screaming in my head. However, my vital signs were not good. My period was throwing my body out of whack. My blood pressure would not go down and my blood oxygen level was alarmingly low. The nurse was giving me oxygen, which I had on all day, and monitoring me closely. I FELT FINE! During the night my oxygen level was so low I heard the nurses talking when they thought I was asleep about sending me to ICU. They couldn't know how my period could wreak havoc on my body coupled with the surgery I had a long road to recovery ahead. I prayed to get better and I asked GOD for help with my recovery I could not die yet I had things to accomplish I wanted to see my great nieces and nephews grow up. Not yet God! I feel asleep praying. In the morning my oxygen level was up and I was doing better.

DECEMBER 17, 2006

The doctor told me that I could go home tomorrow. YEAH!!! I was tired of my body being probed and not getting any rest. Later that day the nurse came to take the IV out of my hand and I could see that it had swollen up. My hand looked like a monster hand or that of a heroin addict when they swell up. I hoped that it would go down and prayed that the scars wouldn't be permanent.

I was now drinking my four ounces of juice every hour. My routine was drinking only apple juice or cranberry diluted with water. I was determined to keep up my routine and I went into my perfectionist mode. I can switch and be a rigid perfectionist or a frivolous shopaholic.

I was in Stage 1 of my diet, which consists of liquids only for two weeks. I had no desire for food and all I wanted to do was regain my strength. I had to introduce vitamins into my system because of the loss of nutrients I was not getting so I took a chewable multivitamin and chewable calcium pills which were nasty but I got use to the taste. I told myself that I needed to take these supplements for the rest of my life because I would not be eating enough food to sustain my body and it was necessary for my survival and recovery.

DECEMBER 18, 2006

I was told that I could go home today and signed the discharge forms. However the doctor came around and told me that because my blood pressure was too high I could not go home. I WAS MAD!!MAD!! MAD!!!!. I wanted out of the hospital!!! When my niece Zyleah arrived to pick me up I told her that I had to stay another day because they wanted to monitor my blood pressure.

I HATE MY PERIOD! I HATE MY PERIOD! I HATE MY PERIOD! My period always has made my body go crazy and I was livid. I was tired of being in the hospital. Not getting any rest because they came around to take vitals for you or your roommate. There was constant activity in the hospital and I wanted to be around family.

DECEMBER 19, 2006

I was discharged today and Zyleah came to pick me up. I was HAPPY! She drove me to my sister's apartment in Yonkers. I had to walk up three flights of stairs and by the time I got to the top I was tired. I needed to sit down and rest. I was glad to be out of the hospital. I knew my sister would baby me and take good care of me while I was recovering because that's what she does. My older sister loves to nurse the wounded bird. I think all of my sisters and I love to nurture others and help out those less fortunate we get it from our mother and grandmother who were nurtures too.

I continued on my liquid diet regime content that the end would justify the means. I tried to drink my protein shake for the first time and it felt like I wanted to puke. I had to lye down for a while. The feeling was the worst I had experienced in my life. All at once I felt nauseous, light headed and drunk. The feeling passed after I lay down for about half an hour and now I know that new things in my system will cause this effect. I have to learn to eat all over again.

DECEMBER 20, 2006

I was able to get out of the house and drive to a nearby mall to pick up a few things by myself. It was great to get behind the wheel and drive myself. I like being independent and while it's nice to be pampered I don't like having to depend on someone to help me. I put on a Depends and got into the Cadillac and went to the mall. I love to shop. I was happy that I could drive and I loved the sense of freedom until I had to pee about fifteen minutes after leaving home.   Thank goodness for the Depends   because I pied in it twice. I sat in the car laughing to myself as I peed in the diaper. This must be what an elderly person feels like. It was a little humbling but I just couldn't make it to a bathroom. The liquids I was consuming were running thru me, which is common on a liquid diet. I went into GNC and brought my protein mix and went home to change my Depends. I had a good night's sleep.

DECEMBER 21, 2006

When I woke up today I was anticipating going to my doctor to have the staples removed from my stomach. I felt good today but I did not want to drive to the office so I took a cab from Yonkers to the Bronx. This was the first time seeing my doctor since the surgery. I was worried that the removal of the stitches would hurt and I braced myself. When the doctor took what looked like tweezers out and plucked the staples out it hurt slightly like a burning sensation but it was bearable and less painful than I thought it would be. Next he covered it with a paper taping to keep the skin together while it heals. Then he gave me a prescription for medication that will prevent gallstones from developing while I heal. He told me that I could go to

Phase 2 of the program, which consisted of pureed foods – baby food basically. I felt good today. I went to the toy store to do a little Christmas shopping for the nieces and nephews after I left the doctor.

The protein shakes no longer make me sick when I drink them.

DECEMBER 22, 2006

I went to Staten Island to stay with my other older sister who has three kids, all school age. I had to rely on Zyleah again to drive the 90-minute trip. I would drive locally. I arrived at night with cups and potions in hand. I had a travel bag that included all my medications, Depends and infant cups because they were the perfect 4oz measurement I needed. I was now taking the gallstone medication twice a day. The medication made me nauseous but because they were capsules I would open them up and pour the powder into the protein shake and blend it all together which made it easier to digest.

DECEMBER 23, 2006

It was my first full day on Staten Island and I slept most of it. I feel as though I need to sleep. I have no energy and no desire to do anything. I just want to be left alone. I don't care that Christmas is coming. I have done my shopping. I don't want anything for Christmas except to have the energy to move about. I feel like I am walking in a daze. I'm able to control my blatter better but I still wear my Depends because it's easier.

I now eat baby food. Breakfast usually consists of farina. Lunch is squash and mashed potatoes and dinner is usually the same.

DECEMBER 24, 2006

CHRISTMAS EVE

I went out shopping with my family shopping to Kmart and Pathmark. I tire easily and had to sit down outside one of the stores and wait for the cab. When I arrived home some diluted apple juice helped me feel better. It wasn't a good day.

Last year at this time I was sitting around drinking homemade eggnog, eating Danish butter cookies and listening to music. However this year I just wanted to rest and I had no desire for sugar.

DECEMBER 25, 2006
CHRISTMAS DAY

I awoke this morning I felt fatigued and sluggish. My energy level was low. I didn't care that it was Christmas nor did I want to open any gifts. I just didn't care. Since I have no children Christmas has no magic for me. My grandmother died around Christmas time and since then it has been a bittersweet time for me. I enjoy watching my nieces and nephews open their gifts and the happy look on their faces when they get what they want. However, as an adult it's just another day. My sister was encouraging me to open my gifts because she bought me a Play station with a Grand theft Auto game so that I could drive and run people over in the game because I always threaten to do so when driving. I also got a Barbie doll because I collect them and gift cards.

After I took a nap I was able to cook lasagna and ham with the help of my nephew Quency but I didn't taste anything. My allergies were bothering me badly but I made it through the day.

DECEMBER 26, 2006

My allergies worsened today. I began to cough and my asthma was bothering. I needed a treatment for my asthma and used my niece's nebulizer. My sister has a cat, which I'm allergic to. I made it through the day and ate my baby food. Breakfast consisted of Farina a tablespoon hour until after which I waited an hour and a half to drink my 4 oz of liquid, diluted juice, then every lunch I had liquid, diluted juice or water. I would drink fifteen minutes before eating to curb the amount I ate as suggested by the nutritionist. Lunch was a tablespoon of baby sweet potatoes and mashed potatoes, no meat. I actually don't eat any red meat. Dinner was usually the same. In between the meals and liquids I had to drink my protein shakes.

DECEMBER 29, 2006

I had to leave Staten Island to go back to Yonkers hoping to alleviate my asthma. My niece and nephew came alone with me. I arrived at my sister's house to find that my oldest niece, her boyfriend and baby were staying there because of hard times. The house was packed but I couldn't go to my house because there had been a flood and the molded smell affected my asthma. I had no home to go to and I had to recover from surgery. I prayed for help.

DECEMBER 30, 2007

I was still eating baby/pureed food. Farina was my breakfast staple. Lunched consisted of a tablespoon of tuna and dinner was a tablespoon of mashed potatoes and some baby vegetables. I was craving a salad badly. I had no cravings for anything accept salad. It was like I had been brainwashed and only wanted healthy foods. I love tofu and have not eaten red meat in about ten years. I ate healthy before my surgery but I binged on sweets and starches, I love bread. I usually ate without thinking about what I was eating or counting calories. I did exercise and became an Aerobics Instructor last year but the pounds kept creeping up on me. I grew up the cute chubby baby sister and have never been thin. My mother dressed me well in chubby clothes that fitted me and were fashionable. When I turned 15 my mother sent me to Elaine Powers, which is equivalent to today's Lucille Roberts to lose weight. I exercised but I still ate. My mother was overweight but she made weight an issue for my oldest sister and me. My weight continued to balloon in high school and by graduation I was about 220 pounds. I never dated in high school and stayed in my books. I made good grades and got a scholarship to college.

<u>DECEMBER 31, 2006</u>

<u>NEW YEARS EVE</u>

I had a doctor's appointment today. I was now 18 lbs. thinner and doing well. I was happy but my energy level was still low and I felt off balance. I'm a Libra and I need balance to function. I had no energy to walk and couldn't stand for long. This didn't stop me from going to get a pedicure, which I do twice a month. I had to look well groomed even if I felt like shit. before the New Year came in. When my nephew woke me it was 12:08am This New Year's Eve would be different because I was ill and mopped around the house with low energy and I felt like a breeze could blow me over. Last year at this time I gathered the family together and provided food and cocktails for everyone and watched them act crazy. But this year I laid on the couch and fell asleep. Happy New Year to me!! Maybe next year it will be better.

JANUARY 1, 2007

The first day of the New Year and I was still not feeling myself. I called a friend to let her know I was okay from the surgery but my asthma was still bothering me. Since my niece was here I had to sleep in the bedroom with my teenage niece and infant nephew. I wanted to go home but the smell was unbearable.

I went to the movies today to see In the Pursuit of Happiness. It was a good movie and inspirational. I drank water at the movies when usually I would have bon bons, nachos with cheese sauce and a slurpy but I was satisfied all the same. I still felt weak and unable to stand for a long period and sitting wasn't too comfortable but I made it.

JANUARY 2, 2007

I'm still tired and working on my strength. Maybe my iron is too low. I had Zyleah bring me some iron pills in hopes that this will help. She was so helpful to me in my recovery. It is important that you have someone to help you thru this process.

I am still eating baby food and it's like no problem to me. My family laughs at me often for eating so little. I wonder what my nieces and nephews really think about my choice to lose weight at this stage in my life. I have always been the eccentric aunt who made decisions that were of no surprise to anyone and they encouraged me in my endeavors and schemes. My family has always stood by me even though they had their issues.

JANUARY 3, 2007

I woke up at 8:30am. The first thing I did was drink my 4oz of diluted juice. After that I fixed my farina, one tablespoon, which took me about 30 minutes to eat. I waited an hour and a

half to drink my water with a twist of
lemon. The next hour I had my protein
shake. In between I took my vitamin and
iron pill. I also had to take my blood
pressure medication, calcium and
medication for gallstones. For the
duration of my life I will have to take
supplements to make up for the limited
food intake and I will have to monitor
my blood pressure for vitamins
deficiencies periodically. Lunch was a
tablespoon of tuna. More liquids,
another protein shake. Liquids. Dinner

was mashed potatoes, stage 1 baby food carrots and flaky fish. I ate about one tablespoon of each. I waited an hour and a half then drank more liquids. ended my day.

I worried that my lack of desire to eat at times would make me sick. I drank plenty but food just didn't interest me. I had no energy to exercise but hoped my rapid weight loss wouldn't leave me excessively saggy. Today I drank more than I ate.

<u>JANUARY 7, 2007</u>

I went to see the doctor and I was down another 17 pounds. He said I was doing great and well on my weight to my target of 175 pounds but I want to be about 165 pounds. He said I could go to Phase 3 of my diet where I can eat regular food. I was happy. I went shopping. I could have my salad. I bought lettuce, tomatoes and low calorie salad dressing. I went home and had my salad for dinner. I could only eat a tablespoon of salad but I enjoyed the two bites.

JANUARY 8, 2007

I followed by usually routine. Breakfast was farina, lunch was salad and dinner was salmon and mashed potatoes.

I walked three blocks to pick up my niece from the bus stop and the walk made me sick. I had to sit down and rest. I can't believe that I still have no energy. I continue to feel sluggish and unmotivated to do anything. I don't even find the opposite sex appealing. I love sex but have no desire for it nor do I want to date. Who am I kidding? I cannot date anyone in my condition.

JANUARY 9, 2007

I began my day the same as usual. In the afternoon I went to pick up my niece at the bus stop and had to run home to go to the bathroom. I don't know why but I shit and spit up at the same time. It was disgusting. Thank God I'm single right now because a man would not find this attractive at all. I can't believe that I put myself thru this. I don't know what the final me will look like or feel like. Will I miss the weight? Will my fat friends hate me? Will men find me attractive? Will I attract a different type of man? I have a lot of questions about this transition and I keep them to myself. I don't really have anyone to talk to about the process or what I can expect. My telephone buddy Vanessa is sometimes helpful when I really need to talk about my concerns because she went thru the surgery. She says that her life changed and she had to change jobs. I know that when I go back to work I want to work in a different borough because I don't want to see the same people and see the look of envy in their eyes or continue to watch them struggle with diets like I did. I have done almost every diet out there; pills, liquids etc. and they all led me to surgery. Diets don't work.

JANUARY 10, 2007

I went back to Staten Island feeling about 65% myself back. I could start exercising. I realized that my thighs were getting thinner. Thank God. They are the biggest part of my body and I hate them. I hate my thighs. I hate my thighs.

I went to the movies to see Stomp the Yard and got my water. I was more comfortable in the movies this time and I felt great today. When I got home I drank some water and I realized that if I drink too fast that I would throw it up. Which I did! I cannot tolerate any beverages that are too cold or too hot. They have to be at room temperature for me to drink them.

JANUARY 16, 2007

This morning I walked my niece to get the school bus, which was about six blocks away from the house. It was hard for me but I didn't feel sick. I had to get out of the house and exercise. I was still feeling weak but I was thinner. I came home winded but feeling comfortable. I continued on my routine of drinking and eating. It feels good to be up and about. I'm coming back to life. At night I got a stomachache and I couldn't move my bowels. I have always suffered from constipation but it had been a week since I went. I called my doctor and he recommended over the medication like ex-lax etc. I went to sleep in pain because the stores in the area that was open only carried Cintroma, which my doctor advised against.

JANUARY 18, 2007

Thank God! I moved my bowels first thing this morning. After taking my niece to school I went to the bathroom again as soon as I came home. I felt relieved. Maybe I just needed to move about to get my bowels moving.

I called my job to find out what papers I had to submit to return to work. I was worried about returning to work and how I would maintain my diet while at work or if I would succumb to the temptations around me.

<u>JANUARY 25, 2007</u>

My girlfriend invited me to an after work party to raise money for the March of Dimes. I was excited to being going out to be among adults and socialize. I put on a pair of slacks that I previously could not fit and felt good. My knee-high boots were loose at the top and I was impressed with me. WOW as I looked at me in the mirror it felt surreal. It felt like I was looking at the me I had always wanted to look back at me in the mirror and now it really was me. I took the ferry into Manhattan and walked to the bus stop. While I waited for the bus in the cold winter night, my stomach began to ache. I felt that I had sat down. When I realized that my bowels needed to be relived I headed back to the ferry to try to make it home. However, holding my bowels is toxic and I get chest pains and feel like throwing up. I made it to the ferry and the next one was in fifteen minutes but as I waited I couldn't hold it anymore and went to the rest room. All at once I started to shit

and throw up. I missed the ferry. Twenty minutes later I emerged feeling relieved but I knew I wasn't finished I caught the ferry home. When I reached home I lay down and went to sleep. I was exhausted. There goes my attempt to socialize.

JANUARY 26, 2007

I awoke this morning and moved my bowels again. Now I felt completed. I was to return to work today but my job requested the original paper work not a faxed copy. I had to call my doctor and have him mail me the original. I was going to take it to my main office but I was feeling under the weather today. I have not been moving my bowels regularly since beginning to eat normal foods. A laxative is needed once a week.

I went to the main office for my job and found out that I should have been at work Monday. Nevertheless, I will start on Wednesday. I spent the rest of the day running errands and enjoying my last day of freedom. Today I found a health food store in Brooklyn, which sold tofu that I had been craving and it was delicious. It was my last day of freedom because tomorrow it was back to work

.<u>JANUARY 31, 2007</u>

I returned to work and got transferred to another borough where I wanted to work. My co-workers were shocked to learn I was not returning to the old position. They were anticipating seeing my weight loss but I had only lost about 30lbs. And I want them to see me in the summer when I hope to be down another 30 pounds.

The first day of work I got up early to eat breakfast oatmeal and pack my lunch. I brought a tablespoon of chili, six crackers and vitamin water. Glaceau Vitamin Water was my saving grace when the taste for water was beginning to make me sick. You can only drink so much water. The Vitamin water has less calories and sugar and the taste is pleasant. I had the same thing for dinner.

FEBRUARY 1, 2007

Another day at work, I have to get used to being around people again. I feel like I have been isolated from society. I have only had contact with my family and my conversational skills have been limited to them. I feel like the women who return from maternity leave after a year alone with their baby. It's a feeling of disconnection and although you are friendly you still tend to isolate yourself subconsciously. Moreover, my co-workers gathered in a room during lunch and ate but I felt self-conscious because they were eating big lunches and here I was with a my small baby lunch having to explain that I can't eat any more than this or I will get sick I ate the same thing as yesterday for lunch because it's easy and I love the tomatoes in the sauce because the taste is like heaven for me right now. I'll work my way up to eating with my co-workers.

FEBRUARY 2, 2007

TGIF and I have my period welcome to the weekend. Today I went to my old office and packed up my stuff after work when nobody was there. The journey from Staten Island to the Bronx took about 2 ½ hours because I did not want to take the train and opted for the express bus instead. I don't like being on crowded trains underground for long periods of time. I checked my voice mail messages and found a message from an ex-boyfriend. I took the number down but I did not call. I don't know if I will call because right now I feel venerable not to mention he left me for another women and cheated on me while we were together. He was a dog but he would do anything for me and give me anything I needed. I want that touch of the opposite sex but I don't want to fall back into bad habits. I've been celibate for seven months and want to make it a year. After I look fabulous I want to be celibate until I marry. I don't know if that will happen because I LOOOOVE SEX!!!!

I had a lunchables for lunch which included turkey, cheddar cheese and wheat crackers. I wanted to try something new. However, the crackers felt like they were tearing up my insides. I won't eat them again. For dinner, I ate the last of the chili.

FEBRUARY 3, 2007

The weekend is here and it is time to try some other foods. Breakfast continues to be one of three things (oatmeal, sometimes with fruit, a scrambled or boiled egg) because it's easy and fast to make in the mornings. Lunch might be a salad alone or with tuna (one tablespoon combined; a slice of deli turkey; or whatever I had for dinner. Dinner today was chicken livers, sweet potatoes and mashed potatoes. It may sound like a lot but I only eat about a tablespoon of each. No butter and lightly seasoned with salt and pepper. Sometimes no seasonings at all taste fine to me. I don't like spicy food and I have always preferred my food a little bland.

<u>FEBRUARY 4, 2007</u>

Today is my mother's birthday and would have been her 77th birthday but she has been deceased for three years. I wasn't sad until my sister reminded me of today. I wonder what my mother would say about me having surgery and losing the weight. She probably wouldn't like it and say why you are doing that to yourself just go on a diet. My mother was obese and had been on many diets herself and knows that they do not work. She was the one who made me obsessive about my weight and appearance. Nevertheless, I wish I could have one more day with her. I was feeling pain on the left side of my lower abdomen. It feels like an obstruction. I have not had a bowel movement as yet and may have to rely on a laxative again.

FEBRUARY 5, 2007

The workweek began again and this will be my first full week back at work. I have no assignment at my work site, which is in turmoil due to many personnel changes. Breakfast was a boiled egg only. For lunch I decided to try a chicken wrap. I could only eat half of the half and I had the remaining half for dinner. In between meals I drink six ounces of vitamin water or regular water.

Today was like the first day, confusion reigns. Breakfast was the same. For lunch I had the half of the chicken wrap and then ate the remainder for dinner

More of the same crap in the office awaited me today. Breakfast included a boiled egg. Lunch was a turkey wrap from Subways, which I ate the same way as the chicken wrap. Dinner was the remainder of the wrap.

FEBRUARY 11, 2007

I went to the doctor for my monthly check up. I have now lost 46 pounds. I like the way my thighs look in jeans and the weight loss is noticeable. The doctor says that I am doing well and my progress is going so well that my next appointment is for two months.

<u>FEBRUARY 12, 2007</u>

The beginning of another workweek. I knew going back to work would be an adjustment for me. Trying to keep on schedule with my eating and drinking and doing your my was becoming difficult but I had to focus and remember my goal. When I went to work and had to go into the field and visit different houses. It had been about three years since I had left my desk and went into the field. It's not easy trying to navigate and find different addresses in an area that you are not familiar with. When I finished for the day I headed home and immediately fell asleep and slept until the next morning. I felt like I had been beat up because I had not been so active in a long time.

FEBRUARY 13, 2007

I called my ex-boyfriend. I couldn't help myself. We chitchatted and he wanted to see me. I wanted him to see what he was missing and to show him that I was just fine without him. I was so in love with him that when the relationship ended I felt depressed for years and did not date because I had no trust for men. I know I need therapy to deal these issues but now my focus is on my weight loss.

<u>FEBRUARY 17, 2007</u>

He called me while I was in Yonkers and said that he was in the Bronx and wanted to stop by. I wanted to see him but I was scared to see him too. I told him he could come by if he wanted to. My sister liked him and she wanted to see him too. She seemed to forget that he cheated on me and brought the girl to the house and left me homeless. My family is strange. But I guess she was only following my lead because I continued to see him after he left me and started living with someone else. I even took him to the hospital when he got sick and almost went into a diabetic coma. YEAH I was STUCK ON STUPID!! He came to my sisters' house and saw me. He was shocked by my size and I told him that I had had surgery so that he would not assume that I was sick or on drugs.

We talked a little and he left an hour later. I didn't have the feelings I once had for him. GOOD!

FEBRUARY 24, 2007

The weekend is here. I decided to drive around the Bronx and Yonkers and found it relaxing to be behind the wheel again. During my recovery I didn't drive because I didn't want to become ill while I was driving. Being on the open road and not having to depend on someone to get around felt great. While in Yonkers I went shopping at New York and Company and found a pair of pants that I could fit. I was elated that the pants fit me comfortable. Then I bought shirts from the GAP. They have a campaign going on with the red T-shirts and I have wanted one since X-mas. I'm most happy about the shopping but this was the first day that I ate out at a restaurant. My family and I went to Applebee's for dinner. I was nervous because I didn't want to be sick. I ordered boneless buffalo chicken and after one I needed water but I can't drink water until one hour after I eat. My mouth was burning but I dealt with it until my side of garlic-mashed potatoes came and eased the burning. I watched my family eat and felt more at ease that my first dinning out experience went well. I didn't feel pressured to eat and it didn't matter to me that everyone around me was eating and sampling until they were full. I had my niece order the Blondie, which is a white brownie with vanilla ice cream and warm topping just so that I could smell it. When I smell the food it's as good as tasting it these days. I love the smell of Cheetos, it's like a high and I get a feeling of euphoria and satisfaction at the same time.

MARCH 4, 2007

I found out that my oldest nephew was incarcerated. He was already on probation and he would now have his first felony offense and face jail time. It hurt my heart to know that he would be locked up like an animal. After watching so many prison movies I was sad to think that he would be incarcerated but I had tried to help him in the past and maybe this is the wake up call he needs. He was attending school and living on his own but he still wanted fast money. I helped to rear him and thought of him as my son since I have no children of my own. You can lead a horse to water but you cannot make them drink.

MARCH 6, 2007

I saw one of my girlfriends who hadn't seen me since my surgery and she thought I looked good. She has lost twenty pounds herself. Since my friends know of my surgery they have all been dieting or contemplating surgery themselves. I feel like the poster child for weight loss surgery. Many people think I was crazy for doing the surgery and say that you just need to eat less and exercise more to get the weight off. I have been on many diet programs and do exercise regularly. In fact I am a certified Aerobics Instructor. Nevertheless, the weight just wouldn't come off. My overeating didn't help. I was a sugar and starch junkie with a slow metabolism. Today my older sister was hospitalized and her two younger children ages 5 and 2 had to be taken care of by the family.

MARCH 13, 2007

I went out into the field again and I was not so exhausted this time. I packed my lunch, snacks and water and continue to keep on my routine. It was my four-month anniversary and I was happy to be losing weight and not eating anything bad for me. I loved my Glaceau Vitamin Waters and thought they were a godsend.

<u>MARCH 19, 2007</u>

I had come into some money and paid off my bills and decided to plan my summer vacations. I planned trips to New Orleans for the Essence Music Festival in July and rented a house in Kissimee, Florida so we could go to Disney World in August.

I brought my 2yo nephew to Staten Island to take care of him for a couple of weeks while one of my nieces took care of the 5yo that was in school. I put my nephew in daycare while I worked. He is a very hyper child and thank god for daycare because by the time I picked him up at 6pm he was ready to go home, eat, take a bathe and go to sleep.

<u>MARCH 24, 2007</u>

I bought a car today!! I was driving in my nephews Cadillac when I saw a Ford Explorer for sale in the Bronx. I stopped and bought the car on the spot. I was elated. Since my first car a Mercury Tracer was hit by a truck I don't want any more small cars and have fallen in love with trucks. Between my nephew being in jail and my sister being in the hospital this is what is needed to bring some joy in my life. I'm going without food and sex I needed some joy.

I decided this month to take a real estate class so that I could make some extra income and not have to work scheduled hours. Every year I picked some new class to attend or a new skill to acquire because I never want to stop learning.

APRIL 8, 2007

It's Easter Sunday. My mother always made a big thing of Easter since we are Catholic. Easter was a big celebration. I remember when I was little she would dress my siblings and me up with hats and gloves for church. Of course patent leather shoes were a must. I continued the tradition and I took my family to the Copacabana for an Easter Party given by a local radio station WBLS. They had live music, food, which we never got, and entertainment for the kids. It was disorganized but it was something to do for the holidays and the kids enjoyed the show.

Tomorrow my classes in real estate begin. I will be going four days a week from 6pm to 10pm. It was an adjustment to go from work to class but I enjoyed learning new things and needed to keep busy so that I didn't think about my nephew or sister. You know what they say an idle mind is the devil's workshop which means that you should keep busy or you will get into negative things because you have no direction or purpose.

APRIL 10, 2007

Thank God my sister came home from the hospital today after being there for about a month. My sister is always ill and is a chronic asthmatic that has never held a job. She receives disability. She is always in and out of the hospital. I know there is a GOD because he always brought her back from the brink of death. She has been in the ICU countless times. I guess her work here on earth is not done.

I waited for the weekend to take her son back home to Yonkers. He is a handful but he is fun and lovable as he always wakes up with a smile and happy raring to go.

I continued to eat the same foods not wanting to stray for fear that I would get sick or throw up. I bought a scale after the surgery and have been weighing myself every day. I know this sounds crazy but I want to know if I need to exercise more or eat less to keep losing weight. It is recommended that you eat six small meals a day to lose weight and take at least 10,000 steps. I also have a pedometer to measure my steps.

MAY 12, 2007

I woke up this morning and decided I needed a change so I went to get my belly button pierced. It was a little painful but bearable. I thought that since the weight loss I needed a little change and I had always wanted to do this but my stomach was too big. I was no stranger to piercings. I have had my tongue, eyebrow and chin pierced in the past.

I weighed myself and I was not 200 lbs yet. This was my goal for the month.

<u>MAY 31, 2007</u>

I was down to 200lbs. It had been five months and I had lost 79 pounds. I was happy. My energy was up and I was feeling good. I couldn't believe it I was on my way to by reaching my goal. I could wear a size 14 down from a size 24.

I took my final for my real estate class and passed it. Go me!

JUNE 1, 2007

I went to Atlantic City for the weekend. I haven't been to Atlantic City in about twenty years. I drove there which was a little scary to be driving a long distance a lone because it was a two-hour drive and I only got lost once. I was going for a conference to receive certifications in Mat Pilates and Weight Management Consultant. It felt good to exercise and be able to get out and socialize with others who are health conscience. (None of my friends exercise). When I arrived for my Mat Pilates seminar we were taught the different techniques and then given a test at the end of the session. At the end of the class I left to find a hotel for the night because tomorrow was another class.

JUNE 2, 2007

Today was the seminar on Weight Management. It was not an easy class and I felt fat in a class of thin toned instructors. Nevertheless, I was going to learn what I needed to pass the test at the end of the session. Tonight, I walked along the boardwalk alone and did a little gambling in the casino. I won a hundred dollars and left. I liked being out. I stayed to myself but I enjoyed being out. I passed a tarot card reader and decided to go in for a reading. She had no shocking revelations nor could she tell me when Mr. Right would come.

<u>JUNE 8, 2007</u>

I took my sister to get her first tattoo and I got a henna tattoo. We took the train into Manhattan and walked around the Village. It was a nice evening and we had a good time.

Now that summer is here I will have to get more clothes. My t-shirts are even too big. I tried on a pair of denim shorts at Kohl's Department Store and I fit into a size 10. WOW! I bought a few summer items in anticipation of my trips in July and August. In July I was going to

New Orleans. Hurricane Katrina had devastated the area in 2005 but the Essence Music Festival was back. I was apprehensive to see the area and a little worried but excited too. Of course I was going with Zyleah. In August I was going with my sister, her three kids, my great-niece and godson to Florida were I had rented a house with a pool. I had planned both vacations in advance and I needed the break.

JULY 2007

I love the summer! The hotter the better for me. Zyleah and I were in New Orleans for the 4th of July weekend to attend the Essence Music Festival. I am in love with New Orleans because you can party in the streets all nights and it's a good time for everyone. I had to adjust to traveling and eating out. I prayed that I wouldn't get sick but my energy level wasn't what I had hoped. I was asleep by midnight and I even fell asleep during one of the concerts after having a couple of sips of liquor. I enjoyed getting away but didn't have energy to party all night like I used to. I didn't even walk down Bourbon Street after the concerts. I was glad that I was able to show her that I appreciated all the help she gave to me during my recovery. I stayed on my diet and ate little. We were able to share plates of food. This was a good month because I was looking good and this was the first summer after my surgery that I could show off the weight loss.

AUGUST 2007

I went to Florida for a week with my family. We had rented a house with a pool and a playroom that had a pool table. We had a ball. I had more energy for this trip than last month. We rented a minivan and drove everywhere. We went to Disney World, Islands of Adventure, SeaWorld and Epcot Center. I kept on my diet and was able to drink a soda without being sick. I even tasted a Slushy. The weather is so hot that all you want to do is stay cool and hydrated.

I ate sandwiches and fruit and stayed away sugar the enemy.

SEPTEMBER 25, 2007

I received a call from my ex-lover who I have not heard from in a year. However, I mailed him a toy car with a note to contact me about a couple of weeks ago. When he finally contactyed me he informed me that he had brought a house upstate and a new car. He says that I will always be in his life and that I must love him. I told him that he could write me out of his life at any time and

J. Camille Kelly

that I like him a lot. Nevertheless, he said that he would maintain contact with me and we would get together soon. I told him that I had changed. His reply was that I always took care of myself and that he was sure that I looked good. I didn't tell him that I had lost weight.

He was used to having sex with a big girl and loved it. Will he still enjoy sex with me? I don't know if we will have sex again?

118

SEPTEMBER 29, 2007

My 14 year-old niece and 12-year-old nephew joined me to perform community service with Boost Mobile Rock Corps. We painted a fence at a local park to earn a ticket for a concert on 10/5/07. We had to give 4 hours of our time to earn the concert tickets. The kids and I worked from 9am-12noon and were exhausted but we were glad that we volunteered and would do it again.

OCTOBER 2, 2007

It's my birthday! Happy Birthday to me! I'm thinner than I have ever been in my life or in high school and loving it. I don't care that I have no boyfriend or haven't had sex in a year. I look good.

OCTOBER 5, 2007

I went to the Boost Mobile Rock Corps Concert at Radio City Music Hall with my 14 year old niece and her 12-year-old brother. It was their first concert and we had a ball.

OCTOBER 12, 2007

I went to the doctor for a check up and I am down to 185 pounds. YAHOOOOOOO! I love the fact that I can fit into a size 10 pair of Levi jeans. The large sizes that I bought at New York & Company and GAP are too big. This winter I'll have to buy all new coats as I wear a size 10 now. I can wear a small/medium top. The surprising thing to me is that when I was bigger I wore only thongs and now all I want to wear is boy shorts. I can wear a size 5/6 in

Hanes underwear. My friends look at me now and say that I look great and shouldn't lose any more weight but for my height this weight still puts my BMI (body mass index) at obese. Wow! At 5'4" I should weigh about 150 pounds to lower my BMI. I think I can do this but what size will I be wearing then. I do see myself losing another 20- 30 pounds.

OCTOBER 17, 2007

I checked my voice mail at work and I had received a message from an old lover who has been trying to reach me. I kind of feel nervous to see him but I know that I have to see him and see if this relationship can progress or should be buried. I wonder if he will like the thin me.

<u>OCTOBER 26, 2007</u>

My nephew is home from jail after spending 9 months away. I am worried that he will not do the right thing and hope that his negative behavior will not affect me.

<u>OCTOBER 27, 2007</u>

I went to a Halloween party at a club, which was sponsored by KISS FM, a local radio station and featured live performances. I dressed as a pirate in a form fitting dress with boots. I looked good but some skinny looking guy only hit me on once. I like my men tall and big (muscular not fat). It was the first time I had been and I think its time that I socialize again. I haven't had a date in God knows when. My last relationship was over six years ago and ended badly leaving me a little jaded and apprehensive about love and men. I'm trying to change myself so that I attract the right men for me. Well this night was a bust as it ended with my car being towed.

NOVEMBER 3, 2007

Today I decided I wanted to go to a club in Manhattan and do some dancing. I danced a little but the music sucked. I got hit on not like before. One male just came up to me and grabbed me around my waist and said that he wanted to get to know me but it wasn't the same as before. This never happened before. I don't like these aggressive tactics and removed myself from him fast. Another male asked me if he could buy me a drink and I declined because I don't drink. I was a little overwhelmed. I haven't been out in so long, is this the way skinny women get hit on? When I was bigger, I had to dance with a guy before I got a drink. It's definitely an adjustment the way people respond to you based on your looks. I mean you see on talk shows that when thin women put on fat suits and go out in public they see that the world is not as friendly to them as when they were thin. Well I'm living that reality. I now have a small waist and a flat ass. Not your typical sister shape.

<u>NOVEMBER 15, 2007</u>

I went to a party given by my job at Tavern on the Green in Manhattan. I saw many of my co-workers from my old office and many of them walked past me and did not recognize me. I loved it!!! They were shocked to see how thin I was and all said that I looked great. My best friend didn't even know that it was me. I think I look the same but because my face is thinner my cheekbones are higher and give my features a new look. One co-worker said that she only recognized me by my eyes. Many male co-workers were shocked and said that I looked great and flirted shamelessly with me. It's kind of a new world for me but I like it.

I was speaking to one of my friends at the party and I told her that I wanted plastic surgery she stated that I was becoming obsessive about my weight loss and talked about it too much. (Only a best friend forever could tell you this) Maybe I am a little obsessive but so what. Maybe she is jealous because she is not skinny. I just won't talk to her about it anymore.

NOVEMBER 20, 2007

I saw an old lover today who I haven't seen in over a year. I didn't tell him about the weight loss. When he saw me he was shocked to say the least. He prefers a sister with meat on her bones and obviously preferred my voluptuous frame. I always thought I was too big, even when he wanted to keep the lights on during sex it made me feel self-conscious. He refused to hug me until he adjusted to my look, which took about half an hour to forty-five minutes. I didn't see it as a big deal. I have known this brother for over ten years. We have both experienced changes in our lives and I thought he would accept the new me with excitement, was I wrong. When I saw him about a year and a half ago he had gained weight and I still accepted him (that's a woman for you). He used to look like the wrestler "The Rock" and now he has a big stomach and no definition to his form but I still find him attractive. He commented about the fact that he could now see my shoulders, which he had not noticed before. (He was too busy looking at my boobs). He commented on the fact that I looked short. My thighs are still full and my breast have deflated some but I'm still a "D" cup. I was a triple D/E cup prior to surgery but, you can always buy breast. He says that he now has a gym in his new house, (which he obviously isn't using) and will go back to working out soon, I hope so. I liked seeing the definition in his body but his broad muscular shoulders are now rounded and because of his weight gain he doesn't look 6'4" tall.

Finally, he hugged me and said that I looked good. Next we went to a bar and had drinks, which we never did, and he introduced me to a couple of people. We then drove around which he never did with my fat ass before which he professed to like. He was treating me differently and I wasn't sure how to take him, we both have to adjust. He joked that he could now throw me around during sex. Yes I gave up my celibacy and it was GRRRREAT!!! I'll see if he calls and I don't know what the future holds for us.

DECEMBER 3, 2007

Today I did field work for my job and the cold weather was like I had never experienced. I felt chill to the bone. I think the extra weight helped keep me warm but this winter appears to be headed for a chiller and I will have to dress in layers like I didn't have to before. When you are a big girl you joke about having insulation well now that I'm thin I'll have to buy a mink.

DECEMBER 4, 2007

It's almost a year since my surgery. I have lost about 95 pounds and can now wear a size 8 that boggles my mind because I now weigh 180lbs. I want to lose another 15 pounds and maintain myself at 165. It's weird that I can wear a size 8 and a little scary. Another 15 pounds could make me a comfortable size 7/8 which blows my mind. I don't ever remember being in the single digit sizes. It's scary and exiting at the same time. The possibilities now before me are great. I don't have to just shop in Lane

Bryant and Ashley Stewart anymore and can shop at any store and find my size. What's funny is now that I have lost the weight it feels that everyone around me is fat and I'm the thin girl. It's even crazier that the average size woman is a 14. Recently, I heard studies that if you are overweight your friends will be also. I guess that means that I have to find some thin friends because all my friends are overweight. It stands to reason that birds of a feather flock together; my mother always said this to me who means I have to be weary of the people I associate with to avoid the temptation to over indulge and regain the weight.

Here we go again my period came down. Now I know why I have been craving salt and sugar. I was able to eat a small bag of chips and 4 cookies. However, I felt sick later. My body rejects food and still makes me ill when I eat sugar. I don't grave sugar but my period throws me out of whack and what I may crave today will make me sick tomorrow.

<u>HAPPY ANNIVERSARY TO ME!!!</u>

I'm where I want to be physically. I am happy with the weight loss but the extra skin is difficult to manage. Because I am bottom heavy, the sagging skin is mostly on my thighs and causes irritation and rashes and makes walking challenging. I need to have a thigh lift. During my last doctor visit I found out that I have a hernia, which is a common result of this surgery. Moreover, when I went to get sterilized (no kids here, I love other peoples children) I found out that my cervix is hanging almost to the tip of my vaginal walls, which makes sitting uncomfortable at times. This means more surgery is in my future. Whoever, thinks that this is a quick fix or a cope out is crazy. It's a process like life. If you want a better or longer life then it's worth the journey.

EPILOGUE

I waited for my body to heal one year after surgery and in 2008 I had my hernia repaired and a tummy tuck at the same time. I also had the excess skin removed from my arms and there is no turkey neck. I am happy with my progress and I hope to have thigh lift and breast lift to complete the transformation to a new me. This may sound extreme but you have to go all the way or not go at all. Emotionally, I have to deal with the new admires and they new me. I have changed on the outside but the inside me remains and I like her and she will remain the same giving, loving, eccentric with a thirst for life and knowledge Good luck to all who choose to embark on the journey I took

ABOUT THE AUTHOR

J. Camille Kelly has received certifications from the American Aerobic Association International (AAAI) and the International Sports Medicine Association (ISMA) in Aerobics, Weight Management Consulting and Pilates. She instructed aerobics classes at the New York City Parks and Recreation Department. She was born in Manhattan and raised in the Bronx. She earned a Bachelor of Arts degree in Criminal Justice from John Jay College of Criminal Justice. She currently resides in Staten Island, New York. This is her first novel.

www.ingramcontent.com/pod-product-compliance
Lightning Source LLC
Chambersburg PA
CBHW072134280526
45788CB00002B/638